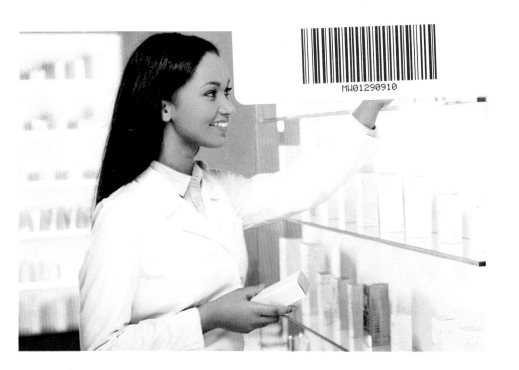

Everyday Natural

Skin Care

This book contains information from a U.S. board- certified dermatologist to assist you with daily skin care and looking your best, regardless of your skin type and your skin history. You will learn crucial steps to daily skin care and preserving or achieving healthy youthful looking skin.

Chapters

Introduction

I have been practicing dermatology for almost 20 years now and after being asked by so many patients and friends every day what to put on their skin or do with their skin, I am eager to teach and share everyone all the latest tips, secrets and myth busters about our skin. There is something for everyone who cares about their skin in this book, whether you are young, old, male or female. It is a must read for anyone and everyone who cares about their skin looking and feeling its best. When you read this book, by all means, skip to chapters that you wish to see first, but be sure and read each topic as they all overlap and connect to one another.

Chapter One

Cleansing, Toning

Why you must cleanse

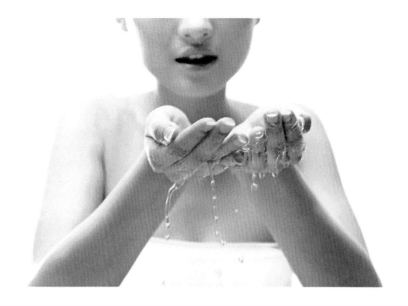

Dermatologists have studied cleansing (cleaning) of the face extensively, and we know that in order to proceed with improving your skin you need to start with a clean palette. Most cleansers are meant to be lathered with water, and applied to your face, and then rinsed off with warm water. There are some cleansers that claim they may be left on the face, but I recommend you rinse off to avoid any residue. I cannot believe how many people I meet that either do not wash their face daily or wash with just water. Just like we cannot clean our dishes with plain water, we cannot adequately clean the oils and dirt off our face with water alone. Cleansing is usually the first step before you apply anything else to your skin.

The home microdermabrasion kit or rotating brushes are best for oily, bumpy, and dull skin free of rosacea or eczema. The purpose of these cleansing tools is to improve exfoliation, which will in turn improve texture and tone in certain skin types. Do not use if you are not willing to disinfect the brush at least once a week and replace brushes monthly or regularly. You may cause more problems with your skin by using them improperly or if you have facial infections or rosacea. See the home device chapter for more information.

There is such a thing as over-cleansing. Dermatologists studied facial cleansing the most in people with acne and we discovered that the best cleansing for acne-prone skin is with your fingertips twice a day and with a gentle cleanser. There are a lot of gentle cleansers available on the market. Years ago, dermatologists studied the ingredients in Cetaphil cleanser and endorsed that cleanser, and then many gentle cleansers copied Cetaphil with their basic ingredients. Research has shown that more aggressive cleansing may give more inflammation to our skin, which may result in more inflamed acne and other rashes.

Toning

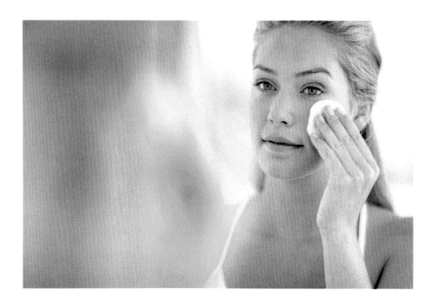

Growing up reading Seventeen magazine, I thought "Sea Breeze" and "Ten O Six" were going to clear my skin and cure my acne. They smelled like they would. The truth is, traditional astringents or oil- control toners are best for very oily skin, and may be too drying for normal or dry skin. Instead the modern toners are meant for balancing pH of our skin so we are less likely to get infections, rashes, and breakouts. Stress, hormone changes, and some diet choices may change the pH of our skin, which in turn alters the flora (bacteria and yeast). Look for gentle toners that restore normal pH for these benefits and apply daily up to twice a day after cleansing. Some dermatologists believe that unhealthy skin pH may be an important cause of acne. Your next step should be moisturizing.

Chapter Two

Moisturizing

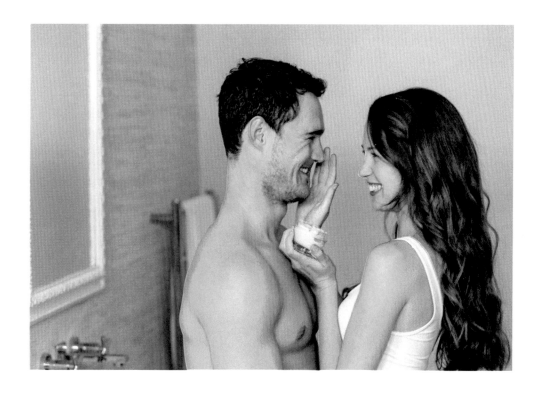

Unless you accumulate shiny oil on your face within an hour of cleansing, you should be moisturizing your face at least once a day, and twice as needed for dryness after cleansing. For acne-prone or oilier skin a lighter "lotion"

moisturizer is best. For dry or neutral skin a cream is best. For the driest skin, an ointment can be used up to one week, and then you should switch to a non-comedogenic cream. Non- comedogenic means it will not make new comedones - blackheads or whiteheads. For sensitive skin, see "sensitive skin" chapter. I prefer to separate the sunblocks from the moisturizer and apply them individually as then you have more control over the ingredients and risk of irritation is less.

Moisturizing is crucial to replace the protective barrier function of the skin when it is compromised, irritated or dried. You can enrich the benefits of your moisturizer by choosing lotions or creams that contain active ingredients to solve your skin problems. If you have a gel or serum with active skin problem solving ingredients, then you will want to moisturize after applying your active gel or serum. For ideas of skin problem solving ingredients, see www.skincreamguide.com.

Chapter Three

Sun Protection

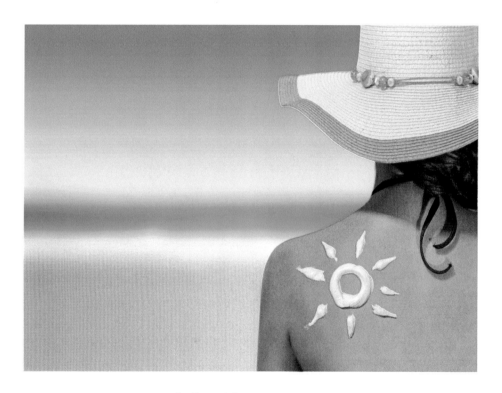

I recommend that if you are going to be outside for more than ten minutes, then you should apply sunblock, minimum SPF 30, to your skin. It is best to choose a mineral sunblock for your face, rather than chemical sunscreens. Mineral sunblocks are: titanium dioxide and/or zinc oxide and function by repelling sun rays off your skin. Chemical sunscreens like avobenzone/Parsol 1789, cinnamic aldehyde, oxybenzone, octinoxate, octisalate and more absorb the sun rays hitting your skin and convert them to heat. This is problematic as it may heat, inflame, or irritate the skin, causing irritant rashes, or worsen brown discoloration or melasma.

Unfortunately chemical sunscreens are rampant on the skin care and makeup market and are often mixed in moisturizers and makeup. When someone is sensitive to sunscreen or gets a rash on their skin after application, it is most likely due to the chemical screens either causing irritation or allergy. Less commonly, some people are sensitive to sun from a disease or medication they take. Women on birth control or hormone supplements will be more sensitive to sun and should be extra cautious to avoid or they may get not only burns, but unattractive brown spots and melasma.

I cannot say enough about the importance of not trusting sunblock to provide full protection, and that it should be combined with use of wide-brimmed hats, long sleeves and shade. Many sunblock manufacturers have elegant face sunblocks that are tinted with a light makeup so they do not look as pasty white. I recommend these tinted blocks for both men and women. They are natural appearing, and do not usually look like visible makeup.

Never trust a cloudy day as a day you can skip your sun protection. I see lots of people in my practice with sunburns on a cloudy day. If you are near water, sand or snow your sun exposure can double or triple due to reflection. At high altitude, for every 1000 feet above sea level, the amount of ultraviolet exposure goes up by approximately 10-12%. For example, if you are at a place that is 5000 feet about see level you will be getting at least 50% more harmful ultraviolet radiation as someone who is at sea level.

Chapter Four

Makeup

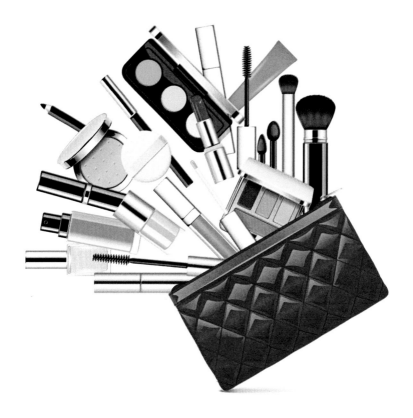

Makeup is not just an art or fashion statement. When makeup is done well it can enhance youth, beauty, wellbeing, and health all at once. When it is overdone or done distastefully it can do the opposite. In this booklet, I am not going to instruct you on all aspects of skillful makeup application but I will offer many practical tips and tricks for anyone applying makeup. Even if you have a shaky hand, or you lack an artist's eye, you still can get good results with knowledge of some basics about makeup.

Makeup should be applied after moisturizer and sunblock for best results. I recommend contouring with a cream or powder base to highlight upper cheeks, mid and tip of nose, brows and temples if you are over 35. Contrary to some contouring makeup kits, do not darken the temples when over 35, as you will just accentuate their aging and hollowness with age.

Avoid applying makeup too thick or it will give an odd, unnatural appearance to your look.

Try to verify your makeup in multiple types of lighting: natural, fluorescent, and soft. Makeup should not be too visible or it will look odd, and repel rather than attract.

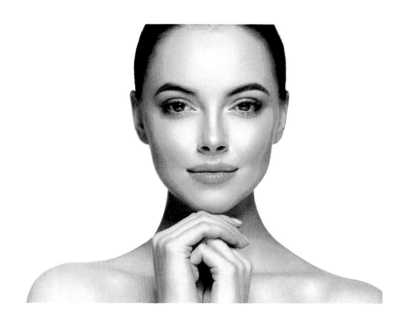

Beauty principles and proportions

Years of research have shown that the most attractive human faces have dimensions that respect the golden phi ratio of 1:1.618. Humans subliminally recognize these perfect dimensions and associate them with beauty. Cosmetic surgeons like myself use this golden phi ratio to determine how best to improve our patient's appearance with fillers, Botox/Dysport, and surgery. Sometimes we will use calipers to verify these facial feature dimensions.

For example, the ratio of the width of the nose to the mouth in the most beautiful men and women is phi or 1:1.618. At home you can respect the golden phi ratios when applying makeup to enhance your beauty. Use darker contours to mask convexities or overly wide places on the face, like a wide nose or wide jaw. Use highlighter to widen eyes if narrow, use darker contour and wear bangs to shorten forehead if tall.

Eyebrows: Enhance eyebrows to draw attention to the eyes and brow, and do not thin and over-pluck eyebrows which can age your look. Thins brows in a woman convey an older, weathered or aged look. While in a man, thin brows can look feminine or less masculine. Avoid drawing or tattooing your brows higher or wider than they naturally grow, or you are likely to have them look less natural. If they are thin, you can use makeup to enhance, or try a prescription like Latisse for eyelashes and off-label for brows.

Corrective/Camouflage makeup: When trying to mask skin wounds, defects, scars, discolorations, and bruises the contour kits as well as the yellow/green/violet correction palettes can be very helpful. It is best to put only thin layers of these types of camouflage makeup to avoid distortion. Many scars and discolorations can be improved with light and laser treatments at the dermatologist's office, so you do not need to suffer in silence.

Lips: Use lipstick to enhance thinned, aged lips, and bring back a youthful and healthy cupid's bow. Eyeliner is helpful to enhance eyes which psychiatric studies have shown are the main focal point when having a person-to-person conversation. Use contour makeup and eyeliner to widen eyes if narrow for a softer, feminine look. Use eyeliner color and eyeshadow color to lighten and soften eyes for a more attractive and feminine look. Studies show lighter eyes score higher when it comes to attraction, and giving the impression of youth, health, and beauty.

Men and Makeup

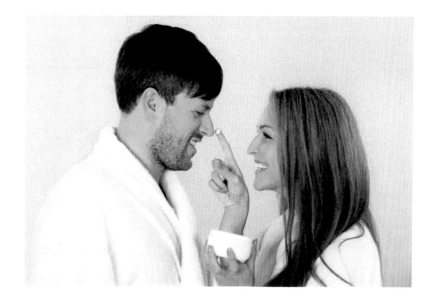

Skin-toned makeup base or foundation is helpful for masking blemishes, red spots, brown spots, and scars whether you are male or female. When men use eye makeup it may feminize their look, which can be desired in some certain art and fashion settings. Men can

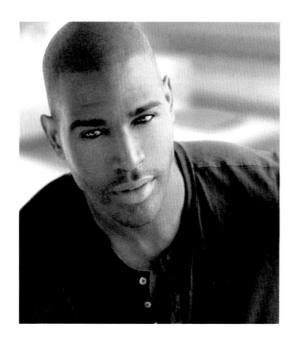

enhance their angles to be more masculine and handsome with contouring makeup, which may be helpful for photographs, and on- camera appearances.

A strong brow and a strong jawline are desirable in men, but an overly strong brow, and closer set eyes can give the impression of anger or threat. As men age, just like women, their temples and mid brow will hollow. Makeup should be applied to highlight these areas, to give the impression that they are stronger or larger than they are.

Chapter Five

Fading Brown Spots and Melasma

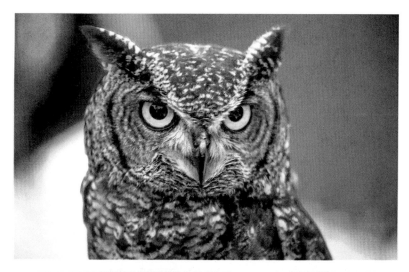

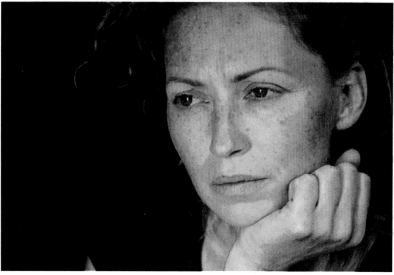

Not all brown spots are attractive as in this owl.

Psychology studies comparing our first impressions of

a person's face when they have lots of brown age spots or freckles vs. not, shows that there is a bias where those with a clearer complexion are believed to be younger, healthier and more competent or reliable at their work.

Before reading this Chapter be sure and read Chapter 3 about sunblocks as sun protection is the number one priority when you have brown spots or melasma of the skin. You must avoid the sun both outside and inside windows in homes and cars to improve melasma and prevent worsening. In addition to avoiding sun, to prevent and control melasma, you must avoid heat to your affected skin as well. Melasma is often triggered and worsened by a combination of hormone changes (like pregnancy), sun, and heat.

There are numerous medications that may cause photosensitivity, or sensitivity to sun: for example, antibiotics, antidepressants, and blood pressure medications. When you begin a new medication, check the packaging for a list of common side effects and look for photosensitivity. Photosensitive skin reactions may result in skin discolorations or worsen melasma, as well as increase one's risk of skin cancer.

Dermatologists refer to common benign brown spots on the skin from sun as "solar lentigos", while melasma is the brown discolored mask of pregnancy or other hormone changes that is worsened by heat and sun. All brown spots on the skin may be worsened by heat and sun or other inflammation.

There are many cosmeceuticals listed on skincreamguide.com that have brown spot or melasma fading power, so it can be tricky to choose.

I suggest that if you are able to afford only one product per month, given they average in price from $40-180, then go with a product that has numerous brown fading ingredients such as: **licorice root extract, niacinamide, kojic acid, soy, AHA or BHA, vitamin C, arbutin, aleosin, alpha lipoic acid, retinol**. While I do not know of a single product with all of those, you can find many with 2+ of those ingredients.

Sometimes, the more ingredients, the more irritating. Be careful not to overdo it, and always test new products on a small area of your skin for a few days before committing. Many of these brown fading creams will irritate in the first week of application and become more tolerable with time or smaller application. In addition, many brown spot fading creams will increase your sensitivity to the sun, but you should be avoiding that anyway.

The Obagi Nuderm system available in some medical offices and medi-spas, has a combination of AHA, and prescription skin lightener - hydroquinone. It is frequently given with the addition of prescription tretinoin, so ultimately has three active brown spot fading ingredients. There are many other popular cosmeceutical grade skin lighteners like SkinMedica's Lytera, and this one is hydroquinone-free but has a combination of effective brown-spot fighting ingredients. There are not enough studies comparing combination products and systems to one another, so I cannot say one is superior to the rest, but just that these combination products and systems tend to work better and faster than a single brown spot fading agent.

The skin lightening agent hydroquinone is available in lower concentrations OTC, but as a prescription at 4%. Hydroquinone is to be used with caution, and never for more than six months or you risk the following side effects: exogenous ochronosis, permanent depigmentation, possible carcinogenicity.

Finally, if you have melasma, you should avoid exposing the affected skin to high temperatures in showers, hot tubs, or saunas. Keep cool or you can worsen the melasma. Chemical suncreens should be avoided as they convert UV radiation to heat when protecting from the sun, and the heat will aggravate your melasma. Instead of chemical sunscreens, choose mineral blocks like titanium dioxide and zinc oxide.

Chapter Six

Controlling Redness and Rosacea

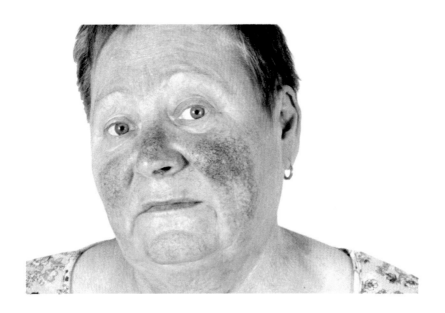

The most important triggers of redness and rosacea to avoid are sun, alcohol, and heat, but many people will develop more redness with certain foods. Spicy foods, alcoholic drinks or foods, temperature-hot foods, and the following foods per rosacea.org:

Liver

Yogurt

Sour cream

Cheese

Chocolate

Vanilla

Soy sauce

Yeast extract

(bread is OK)

Vinegar

Eggplant

Avocadoes

Spinach

Broad-leaf beans

and pods,

including lima,

navy or pea Citrus

fruits, tomatoes,

bananas, red

plums, raisins or

figs

Foods high in histamine

To battle the redness at home, you must avoid irritants or exfoliators on your skin like home microdermabrasion devices or rotating brushes or abrasive cleansers. In general, with rosacea, your skin is more sensitive and you should avoid heavily medicated cleansers meant for acne. You should also avoid chemical peels. Choose gentle, hypoallergenic skin cleansers and moisturizers. It is important to moisturize and maintain the skin barrier as explained in Chapter two.

Try cosmeceutical ingredients known for calming inflammation or fading redness like: aloe vera, niacinamide, licorice, green tea, feverfew, colloidal oatmeal, allantoin, gingko biloba. On skincreamguide.com you can find an A-Z guide of ingredients like these with options for good brand name products containing them. I recommend you choose a product that has a combination of more than one active cosmeceutical ingredient listed for the best results.

Sometimes rosacea may worsen and involve infection of the skin with skin mites. This type of rosacea will usually present with itchy or painful pimple-like bumps or pustules, and is best treated by your dermatologist with prescription topical and oral medications.

Chapter Seven

Controlling Acne

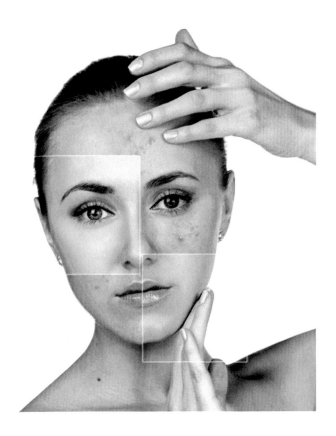

As a teenager with acne, you need a daily routine to best control the acne, and it should include and respect all the steps detailed in Chapters one through six. If your acne is mild or even moderate, you may do well with home steps and remedies and not even need prescriptions. Some of those steps have already been explained in previous chapters like proper cleansing, and sun protection and brown and redness fading, so please go back and read those chapters first. Teens with acne should choose a gentle skin cleanser and moisturizer, and mineral sunblock.

Unfortunately acne is not just for teenagers. Adult acne tends to be lower face, neck and body located. Adult acne is more likely to be secondary to hormone changes, stress or diet factors.

Both teenagers and adults with acne should avoid a high glycemic diet which has been linked to more acne on the skin. In addition, skim or fat free milk should be avoided as it has also been linked to worse acne. Whey protein supplements need further studies regarding acne, but limited small studies showed a link, so I would avoid whey protein as well. Finally, if you have oily scalp or dandruff, then you may have pityrosporum or yeast acne which will not respond to the typical treatments but may improve at home with use of dandruff shampoos to the scalp and skin. This yeast acne is typically seen as small, superficial, pink bumps on the face that may continue into the hairline and into the scalp.

For daily acne control whether you are a teenager or adult, benzoyl peroxide, salicyclic acid, and now Differin gel are the most commonly available treatments without a prescription. Differin gel was the first retinoid to go over the counter, and is an excellent first-line acne medication for mild to moderate acne. It is possible and safe to try these medications along with a natural acne remedy for better results. Choose serums, lotions or gels that contain the following acne-fighting natural ingredients: **aloe vera, niacinamide, licorice root extract, feverfew, vitamin C, green or black tea, witch hazel, tea tree oil**.

Chapter Eight

Controlling Eczema or Dry Skin

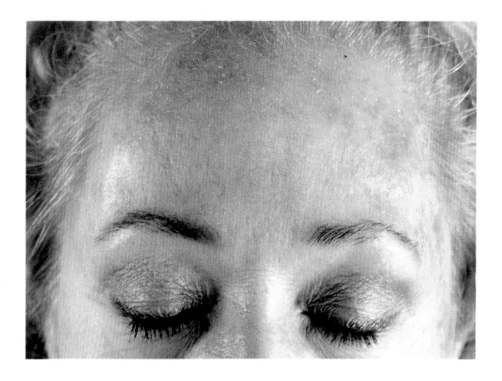

    You must read Chapter Two before this Chapter so you understand basic steps of moisturizing as this is crucial to prevention and control of dry skin or eczema. Some people with eczema, especially when it runs in families may have deficiencies of skin lipids and proteins, so daily use of moisturizers that supplement with these is crucial to getting their eczema under control. If your skin does not have all the necessary components, it will not properly perform its function as a barrier and allow for more infections, and allergies. This is why we tend to see more infections and allergies in people with dry skin and eczema. If you are wondering if you have eczema or psoriasis, it is best to see a dermatologist to clarify.

Dermatologists understand that if your eczema is moderate to severe, then you have a significant chance of having allergies to some skin product ingredients and other allergies to foods or things in our environment. With this type of eczema, it is best that you get tested for allergies with the help of your dermatologist and that you always test new skin products on a small area of your skin for a few days before committing. With all forms of eczema, it is best to choose skin products that are hypoallergenic, fragrance-free, dye-free.

If your dry skin is very flaky and decorates your clothes with white debris, then try moisturizing daily with an exfoliating skin cream that contains and AHA, BHA, or LHA. These are different types of hydroxy acids that will help shed the dead skin cells faster so they do not end up on your clothes. A monthly chemical peel at home, spa, or doctor's office may help your dry skin too and can be done in addition to the home remedies. The following are common side effects of exfoliating skin treatments: increased sun sensitivity, temporary pink color or redness enhanced in the skin, itching or burning sensations during or after application.

I have seen many people over the years who come into my office thinking they have just dry skin, but it turns out they have an infection or a dermatitis like allergic contact or seborrheic. To verify what is causing your dry skin, it is best to see a dermatologist.

When choosing skin creams for dry or eczema-prone skin, always avoid fragrances and dyes, and look for the following natural ingredients: **ceramides, omega fatty acids, evening** primrose oil, sunflower seed oil, linoleic acid, dimethicone, niacinamide, mineral oil, glycerin, urea, chamomile, aloe vera.

Chapter Nine

Fighting Wrinkles and Aging

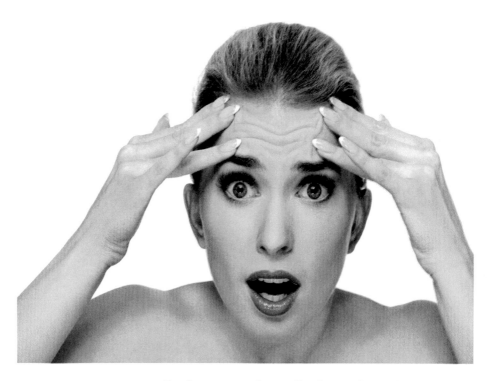

You must read Chapter Three before this chapter to understand how to protect best from sun. Many wrinkles in the skin could be prevented with lifelong sun avoidance. Get your extra vitamin D from diet and supplements and not the sun. Did you ever notice that darker skinned people seem to age more gracefully with fewer wrinkles? Look at Oprah Winfrey. Does she look over 60 to you? Darker skin is better protected from sun damage by the presence of more melanin. Other than that aging skin changes should be the same as a fair skin type.

   While we cannot completely stop our skin from aging, we do have measures that can delay and lessen aging changes. First we need to understand why we get wrinkles. Wrinkles form with age from a combination of loss of structural elements like collagen, elastin, and hyaluronic acid and loss of underlying fat and bone structure. Sun exposure, chemicals, toxins, and stress will hasten loss of these structural elements. In addition, as we age our skin metabolism and the ability of the skin to renew itself slows. Many scientists believe that aging changes are partly secondary to oxidation at a cellular level and that antioxidants offer some protection from this.

   To delay and lessen the aging changes of our skin at your home, I recommend sun protection, daily use of DNA repair ingredients, antioxidants and growth factors. Look for the following anti-aging ingredients in your skin products: **retinol, green tea, soy, curcumin, silymarin, pycnogenol, vitamin C, coenzyme Q10, grapeseed, redox signaling molecules, peptides, growth factors.**

Chapter Ten

Sensitive Skin

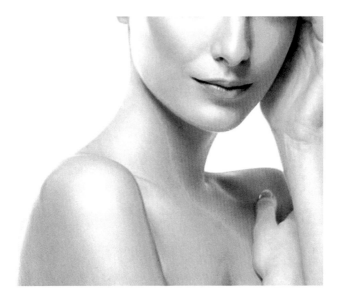

If you have sensitive skin due to eczema or rosacea, then please read the chapters devoted to those subjects as well. When your skin reacts easily to products, good or bad reaction, it could be described as sensitive. Women more often describe their skin as sensitive than men. Sometimes what you thought was sensitive skin is really just dry skin or eczema, so please review Chapter 8 as well.

Cosmeceuticals are skin products that have function that lies somewhere in between a cosmetic and a medicine grade product. Incorporating cosmeceuticals into your daily skin care regimen when you have sensitive skin should be done with caution. Many herbal ingredients are irritants or allergens to sensitive skin. It is wise to start

with products that do not contain many ingredients and test them on a small are of your skin first, such as the inside of your wrist or the side of your face by the ear. Test for a few days before applying to a larger area of your skin.

For the most sensitive skin types, I recommend the following skin care lines, not in any particular order: Cetaphil, CeraVe, Vanicream, True Lipids, and Aveeno. If these products still cause irritation or rash, then white petrolatum, True Lipids ointment, Vaseline or Aquaphor ointments may work daily for body and occasionally on the face. Ointments are the most moisturizing and are not recommended on oily skin areas for more than a few days or acne may occur.

Cleansing is still important when you have sensitive skin. You should gently cleanse your face before applying your lotion or creams or makeup. Cleanse gently with fingertips lathering a liquid cleanser and avoid using wash cloths or rotating brushes. There are many gentle face and body cleansers available that work for this purpose. Cetaphil cleanser is one of the most studied and trusted by dermatologists.

With sensitive skin, try using creams rather than lotions as creams tend to be less irritating. Avoid gels which are the most drying unless you follow it immediately with a soothing cream. Serums have become popular in recent years and they tend to be liquid or oily, and often tolerated well by all skin types, depending on their active ingredients. Some people experience acne flare-ups with vitamin C serums.

With sensitive skin, it is best to use only

mineral makeups and physical sunblocks rather than chemical makeups and sunscreens. Never cleanse your face more than twice a day if you are sensitive.

When choosing skin products to help rejuvenate sensitive skin, consider alternatives to retinoids which tend to be irritating, such as the following examples: **stem cell growth factor cream (SkinMedica TNS, NeoCutis), antioxidant-rich cream (Skinceuticals), peptides (Regenerist), redox signaling molecule serum (ASEA)**

Chapter Eleven

Climate and Skin

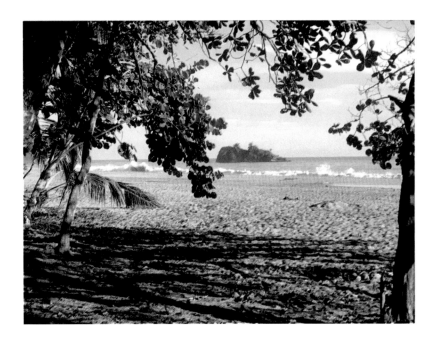

I would like to review some key points about weather or climate and our skin, as many of my patients will tell me that they develop problems seasonally or when they travel. Of course, there are other factors to keep in mind that can affect the skin seasonally or when traveling beyond weather such as diet changes, stress, activities, changes in products. If you keep in mind how weather may impact your skin it will help you better choose your daily skin regimen. We can think we know our skin based on a "skin type" or other unproven theory about how our skin behaves or based on the fact that we have a skin problem like acne or rosacea, but throw yourself into a different climate and what you thought you knew will probably change.

If you live in a hot, humid place like Florida or near the rainforest in central or South America you may not suffer from as many dry skin problems as someone who lives in a dry place like Arizona or the Rocky Mountains. If you have a wet season or dry season, then your skin will be more wet or dry, during those respective seasons. In addition, hard water is believed to be more drying to the skin, then softened water.
There are studies that have shown that oily skin may get more oily in humid environments.

As a dermatologist, I do see more eczema and dry skin complaints in the winter, which is cold and dry where I practice. Though sometimes I will see a swimmer or athlete who has their eczema worse during the summer swim season.

You can try and modify your house environment with air humidifiers or air dehumidifiers or water softeners to help your skin look and feel its best.

Chapter Twelve

Home Devices For Skin

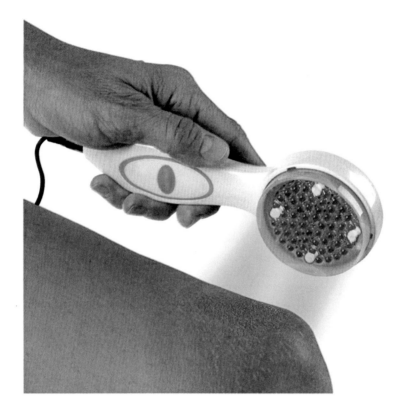

We are seeing all kinds of hand-held devices for home use that promise to improve your skin. There are home rotating brushes and microdermabrasion devices for exfoliating rough or acne-prone skin. There are home lights for fighting acne, removing hair, and rejuvenating. I have seen and tested many of them, and understand their science and have seen the research (or lack thereof) to support their claims. While they are helpful, they are not as powerful as even some creams, lotions, serums that have been discussed in this e-book and can be used at home. Home skin treatment devices are generally not as powerful as in-office laser and light treatments, as if they were, they would be quite unsafe to have in the home.

As of 2017/18 be warned about the rotating brushes. My dermatology colleagues and I have seen and agreed that certain forms of acne and peri-oral dermatitis will worsen with those brushes. This is because such forms of acne, rosacea and peri-oral dermatitis really are due to infections - bacterial or yeast - and such a brush will just spread the infection. In addition, people with a tendency towards allergy and sensitivities may also worsen with the brushes. People with simple comedonal acne (blackheads and whiteheads) or mature adults with just dry skin and wrinkles, usually tolerate and may benefit from the brushes. There is very limited clinical data to support their use. To verify if you have skin appropriate for the brushes, it is best to see an experienced dermatologist.

The new acne home light treatment devices contain blue light which is believed to kill acne-causing bacteria, and red light which is believed to calm inflammation. This is promising technology that is an attempt to simulate the much stronger in-office versions, which actually have research data to prove their efficacy. At present, the home acne lights are not as effective or efficient at controlling acne as the more powerful in-office blue and red lights. For example, to achieve the same improvement in your acne at home, one would have to use the home light treatment twice daily or more, while the in-office treatment can be done once a week. I look forward to clinical studies that compare the two.

The home laser devices are in general marginally effective, as they do not carry the adequate power to execute their treatment goals both efficiently and effectively. For example, the home hair removal laser devices. In order to keep them safe for home use, the low energy is marginally adequate to effectively kill the hair roots. There is the risk that this low energy will stimulate more hair in some people. This phenomenon has been reported when the in-office lasers are used at lower energy. The home rejuvenating, wrinkle-fighting devices may help marginally but with lots of repeat use (multiple times a week), time and effort.

 For male or female pattern balding or hair loss, the home hair regrowing light or laser devices have some success. Studies are showing that these devices, while helpful, are not as effective as oral medications for men like oral Propecia/finasteride, and topical medication like Rogaine/Minoxidil solution. I recommend these devices as an adjunct to the other treatments. Where Propecia is not recommended for women, these home devices along with minoxidil solution may be helpful.

Regarding the safety of these devices. We have many years safety experience with the higher strength in-office versions of these devices, so the lower energy versions are unlikely to pose any harm as well.

ABOUT THE AUTHOR:

Karen Stolman, M.D. is a board-certified Dermatologist in the United States, practicing Dermatology and Dermatologic Surgery since 2001.

Dr. Stolman is also the author of
www.skincreamguide.com and www.skinality.com

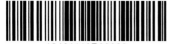

Made in the USA
Lexington, KY
31 October 2018